NSL

Body Wrap

Training Manual

NSL Body Wrap   - Copyright © 2014 by Chrysalis House Publishing

Chrysalis House Publishing

Louise Prunty

Lower Ground

7 Newton Place

Glasgow

G3 7PR

United Kingdom

publishinguk@me.com

www.chrysalishousepublishing.com

Introduction to NSL Wrap.

Thank you for choosing NSL Wrap as your body wrap product. NSL is a 100% natural balm with excellent inch loss results and completely based on nature.

An excellent treatment for beauty and holistic therapists / salons to offer and also a very popular Spa treatment.

This manual is not intended as a replacement for wrap training but as a learning aid for students or used in classroom based training.

If you are already trained in wraps and wish to take a free NSL conversion course please contact info@ctacademy.co.uk

Useful Contacts:

www.nslwrap.com
Brand Owners: www.ctacademy.co.uk
Email: info@ctacademy.co.uk

On completion of your training you will be able to:

1. **Prepare the work area for treatment**

2. **Carry out a full consultation and plan treatment with your client**

3. **Clearly and accurately explain the benefits, contraindications and contra-actions.**

4. **Understand and be able to provide effective NSL body wrap treatments**

5. **Provide accurate and clear aftercare advice to your client**

1: Preparing the work area for treatment

The work area should be prepared in advance of the client's arrival and must be safely set up (free from hazards such as trailing cables, spillages etc) and hygienically clean (work surfaces sanitised, new towels for each client, treatment waste from previous treatments correctly disposed of).

The room should be comfortably, but not excessively, warm. Lighting should be bright enough to allow the therapist to work safely, but low enough to provide a relaxing ambience for the client. Suitable background music can help to create the desired atmosphere .

As products naturally have a sent, it's advisable not to use scented candles or air fresheners in the treatment space (remember, clients may be sensitive to chemicals contained in air fresheners and synthetic perfumes in candles).

This is especially important with NSL wrap, as the products are 100% natural and 96% organic – remember that this may be the reason the client has chosen NSL over other brands on the market, so the treatment environment should be as free as possible from synthetic, chemical – laden products.

The trolley or work surface should be set up with all necessary product and consumables in advance of the client arriving. This will include your NSL kit, consultation form and pen, spatulas and bowls, tissues, tape measure and any disposable clothing items for the client if using these. A lined, lidded pedal bin for hygienic disposal of treatment waste should be nearby.

The treatment couch should be dressed with clean towels or drapes and freshly covered pillows and bolster for each client. A thermal blanket is optional and can increase temporary inch loss via loss of fluid during treatment. Couch roll if used must be changed for each client and disposed of correctly after treatment.

Drinking water should be available for the client, and a chair (not a therapy stool) should be ready for the client to sit on during consultation.

2: Carry out a full consultation and plan treatment with your client.

An example of **a full consultation sheet** is available at the end of this section.

This provides you with the basis for a discussion with your client:

- to establish whether the treatment is safe and suitable for them

- to create a rapport with the client

- to allow time to fully inform the client of what to expect from treatment and to answer any questions they may have.

- To plan and agree on treatment aims and how to proceed.

This must be carried out thoroughly in advance of the first treatment, and you should allow extra time for this when making the appointment. At follow-up appointments, you should check that there are no new health conditions or **contra-actions** from previous sessions that may **contraindicate** treatment and record this, along with a client signature that your notes reflect the discussion accurately. Contraindications and contra-actions are covered more fully later in this manual.

A contraindication is a sign or condition that means that it may be unsafe to proceed with treatment or that treatment may be restricted.

A contra-action is a reaction that occurs either during or after treatment.

Consultation methods

Consultation is essentially a fact-finding exercise , and we can find out information about our client and his/ her needs and expectations via a range of methods. Some of these are explored below.

1. **Observation** : When your client arrives, notice their posture. Are they standing tall with relaxed shoulders? Slouching ? Do they appear tense? Posture can give us clues about a client's mood or attitude as well as an indication of areas of the body that may be tense or tight and perhaps need some additional attention during some treatments.

   Posture can also change our body shape and appearance (this is particularly of note at the measuring stage of preparation for treatment – clients may be self conscious and apprehensive about being measured , and may tend to straighten up and suck in the tummy when the tape appears! Here, it's important to ask them to relax to get an accurate measurement as a baseline to evaluate post-treatment results)

   Think about someone you believe is confident. This can be a friend, family member, celebrity.. anybody who seems comfortable in their own skin . What is it about the way they present that makes you see them as confident? Note down some of these things.

   You may have included such things as good eye contact, relaxed, open body language (no folded arms or crossed legs, or shoulders held high and tight) , a friendly smile - we recognise these signals from other people and interpret them in our day to day life, and it's important that we do this in our working lives as therapists too.

   Observation can give us clues as to whether a client is apprehensive and needs some gentle reassurance, as well as telling us about skin type and condition and even client health and wellbeing.

   Your own posture and non-verbal communication is vital here. Your body language should be open - no crossed legs or folded arms- and relaxed , with appropriate eye contact (not staring at the client, or looking away too often) You should be aware of positioning during consultation - ensure the client is not " hemmed in" by your seat , and sit at a slight angle to the client rather than directly opposite. Leaning in very slightly towards the person indicates interest in what they are saying.

2. **Questioning and listening.** This consultation technique allows us to find out the specific information required to establish whether it is safe and in the client's best interests to proceed with treatment as well as to find out a bit more about the client's lifestyle to allow us to best tailor treatments to their needs.

The consultation form is a tool for carrying this out , and includes two **types of questions – open and closed.**

Closed questions (for example, "are you pregnant?") can be answered "yes" or "no" while **open questions** (such as "what do you hope to achieve from this treatment?") invite a more detailed response from the client. Closed questions are used in the health check section of the consultation to establish whether certain conditions which might affect or rule out treatment are present – however, the therapist should be prepared to follow these up with an open question and not merely stick to the layout of the form. For example, if a client answers yes to any of your closed questions on health (for example , to " have you ever had a thrombosis?") then this should be followed up with "when was this? " , questions about any ongoing effects the clot may have had on health , any medication prescribed and so on. This helps give us a fuller picture and lets us as therapists make a fully informed decision on how and if to proceed. If there is anything you are not sure about, ask further questions to ensure you fully understand what the client is telling you.

Listening is vital! Listening well and effectively is just as important as being able to express yourself clearly verbally. Hearing what is being said and taking it into consideration forms the basis of your consultation and treatment planning.

Active listening is when we listen attentively to someone who's speaking, and show that we are doing this. We show this by nodding or verbally indicating that we're listening ("yes", "OK") where appropriate, not interrupting, and summarising and confirming what the person has said after they have finished speaking. For example:- a client tells you she eats a lot of junk food, snacks a lot during the day , and has gained a lot of weight . She says she doesn't exercise much, but wants to start going to the local gym, and booked this treatment as a kick-start to a new eating and exercise regime. When she's finished speaking, you may sum this up as " So, you want to have this treatment to help to motivate you to start a healthier diet and more active lifestyle? " and wait for her to confirm . This shows you have listened carefully, understood what she was saying, and summarised it – you have also used positive language and framed this as working towards a healthier lifestyle overall rather than just to lose excess weight.

Planning treatment

Based on the information you've gathered both through observation and discussion with the client, you can now agree with the client how you will proceed with the treatment. Here you can inform the client of how you propose to carry out the treatment (agree which parts of the body you will target, what methods you will use – for example you may choose to use dry brushing rather than a scrub to boost circulation - what you would recommend as a follow up (such as perhaps a course of six treatments, specifying the timescale) Give your reasons for your recommendations and ensure that the client is in agreement.

Signatures: ensure that both you and your client have signed and dates the appropriate areas of the form before proceeding – this indicates that you have discussed the options and that the client has given full information , understands how the treatment will be carried out, and gives informed consent for this.

Keeping records:

- It is important to keep accurate records securely in line with data protection legislation and to maintain confidentiality.
- Information must be accurate and relevant to your needs
- You must comply with individual's requests for information that you are holding on them and failure to do so means you are contravening the Data Protection Act

For further information:

Data Protection Register, Springfield House, Water Lane, Wimslow, Cheshire. SK9 5AX

For **follow up appointments**, it is not necessary to carry out such a detailed consultation, but you must check that there are no new health conditions that may affect treatment at each appointment, check for contra-actions following the previous treatment, and record this information, with client signature that it is a true account.

NSL wrap consultation form

The following information is required for your safety and to benefit your health. Whilst NSL Wrap is totally safe when administered professionally by a trained therapist there are certain conditions which may mean the treatment is not suitable or may require special care. The following details will be treated in the strictest of confidence. It may however, be necessary for you to consult your GP before any treatment can be given.

Date of Consultation:

Personal Details

Name:

Address:

Tel No: Daytime: Mobile/Evening:

Date of Birth: Occupation:

Medical Details

Name of Doctor: Surgery:

Address

Tel No:

Do you have/have you ever suffered with any of the following conditions?
(Please give dates and details)

High or low blood pressure	Y	N	
Heart condition	Y	N	

Kidney infection	Y	N	
Thrombosis	Y	N	
Varicose veins or phlebitis	Y	N	
Dysfunction of the nervous system	Y	N	
Recent injury or surgery	Y	N	
Any current infectious condition	Y	N	
Blood disorders	Y	N	
Arthritis	Y	N	
Diabetes	Y	N	
Epilepsy	Y	N	
Asthma	Y	N	
Skin diseases or disorders (inc. sunburn)	Y	N	
Recent haemorrhage	Y	N	
Abdominal or digestive complaint or hernia	Y	N	
Do you have any serious conditions such as cancer or tumours?	Y	N	
Do you have any recent scar tissue/ bruises/ open cuts/large moles/ lumps/other swellings?	Y	N	
Do you suffer from any allergies	Y	N	
Do you have liver disease?	Y	N	
Female clients: Is it possible that you may be pregnant?	Y	N	
Do you have a contraceptive implant ?	Y	N	

Current medical treatment:

Current medication (list dosages):

GP referral required:	Yes ( )	No ( )	
Clearance received:	Yes ( )	No ( )	Date: _____

General State of Health and Lifestyle

Do you smoke?	Yes ( )	Average per day	No ( )
Do you drink alcohol?	Yes ( )	Average weekly consumption	No ( )
How many glasses of water do you drink daily?			
How would you describe your diet?			
Stress levels:	High ( )	Medium ( )	Low ( )
Sleep pattern:	Good ( )	Average ( )	Poor ( )
Do you exercise regularly?	Yes ( )	No ( )	
Details :			

Have you ever had a body wrap before?	Yes ( )	No ( )
If yes, please give brief details of previous treatments and outcomes:		
What do you hope to achieve through this treatment?		

Client Declaration

I declare that the information that I have given is true and correct and that, as far as I am aware, I can undertake treatment with this therapist without any adverse effects. I have been fully informed about contra-indications and possible contra-actions, checked with my health care provider where required, and am willing, to proceed with the treatment.

I agree to report any changes in my health as they arise.

I understand that my body wrap treatment is for relaxation and to assist with the release and elimination of toxins and waste from the body, and that the anticipated inch loss results vary with each individual..

Client's signature:	Date:
Therapist's signature	Date:

Client initials: ....

Area	Initial measurement	Post treatment measurement	Difference
Right calf			
Left calf			
Right thigh			
Left thigh			
Hips			
Lower abdomen			
Waist			
Upper abdomen			
Chest			
Right upper arm			

Left upper arm			
Overall result			

Treatment number: Date:

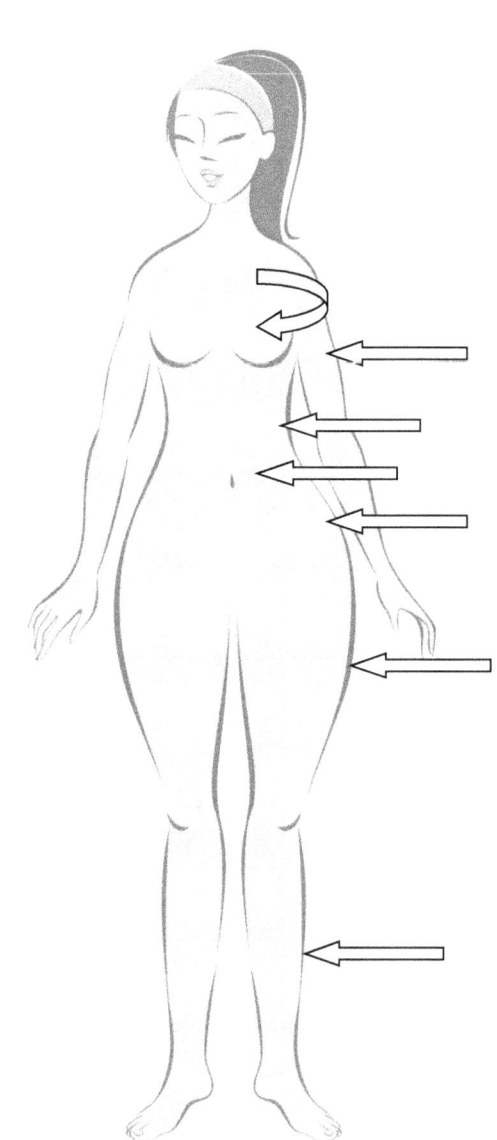

3: Clearly and accurately explain the benefits , contraindications and contra-actions

The benefits of NSL wrap

:

- **Uses 100% natural, 96% organic products** – the balms, scrubs and oils are free from harmful synthetic substances and are carefully formulated to produce maximum results. **See the following pages for ingredients and properties.**

- **Works in two ways to produce inch loss** - promotes lipolysis (this is the breakdown of fat stores – lipids are hydrolysed into fatty acids and glycerol which are carried through the body and processed as waste) , and also operates in a similar way to inch loss wraps which reduce fluid in the body . This double action means NSL produces excellent short- and longer-term results.

- **Hydrates** and improves skin condition

- **Boosts blood and lymph circulation** , carrying nutrients to the skin more efficiently and removing waste more effectively.

- **Promotes detoxification of the body**

- **Brightens skin through promoting desquamation**

- **Induces relaxation of tense muscles**

- **Home use products are available to enhance treatment effects between appointments**

NSL Body Wrap - Suitable for all body types. Even slim clients can lose inches.

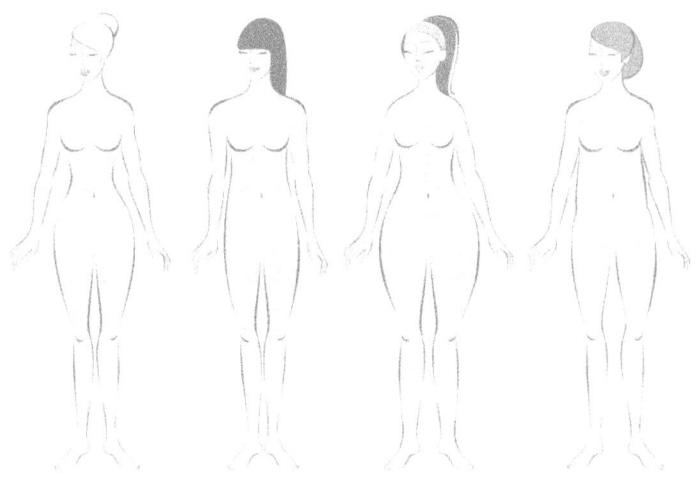

Ingredient	Information and properties
Organic Refined Shea Butter	Hydrating and moisturising ; healing properties via its high content (up to 65%) of cinnamic acid esters, a naturally occurring anti-inflammatory, and 5-10 % phytosterols . These are known to be active in stimulating formation and growth of new cells. Sourced from the Karite or Shea tree nut, so avoid use where there is known nut allergy.
Organic Unrefined Cocoa Butter	Nourishes, protects, moisturises and firms skin. Contains Vitamin E .Has antioxidant properties. Sourced from the seeds of the Cacao tree.
Organic Unrefined Coconut Butter	Adds body and good glide to the product, and keeps skin hydrated during the wrap process. High in lauric acid, and has antifungal and antibacterial qualities.

Ingredient	Information and properties
Organic Pumpkin Seed Oil (cold pressed)	High in vitamins A, B2, B3, beta-carotene and potassium, zinc (which produces a lifting effect) and magnesium. Also contains Omega 9, 6 and 3, and is very useful in facial, abdominal, thigh and breast lifting and firming preparations.
Organic Sunflower Oil (cold pressed)	The oil used in this product is very high in lecithin and oleic content (omega 9)
Organic Ginkgo Tincture	Revitalising, stimulating, firming and has strong antioxidant properties. Ginkgo has been found to stimulate circulation and is therefore good for bringing nutrients to the skin and improving condition and appearance. Very toning and stimulates lipolysis. Sourced from the Ginkgo tree.
Organic Ginseng Tincture	Toning, revitalising and strengthening; stimulates the metabolic activity of the body and has lipolytic properties.
Mullein Oil	Contains tannins, vitamins and minerals, as well as useful levels of elastin, a tissue protein that keeps skin taut and flexible. This helps retain moisture in the skin and can refine the surface texture. Derived from plant sources.
Passionflower Oil (cold pressed)	Stimulating and rejuvenating, with a high essential fatty acids content – high in Omega 3,6 and 9 . Plant derived.

Jojoba Wax	Nourishing, protecting and softening to skin, this is a vegan-friendly alternative to beeswax from a plant rich in nutrients and vitamins.
Remodelling Intense	Formulated from coconut oil and Spilanthes Acmella flower extract, this active ingredient helps to restructure and sculpt the body, firming and smoothing the surface of the skin . Promotes lipolysis.
Rosemary extract	Antioxidant
Rosemary essential oil	Antioxidant, toning, diuretic – extracted from the flowers of the plant via steam distillation. Not suitable for use in pregnancy or people with epilepsy or hypertension.
Juniper Berry essential oil	Diuretic, stimulating and lipolytic; used to help combat cellulite and to promote lymphatic drainage. Not suitable for use in pregnancy or where there is kidney disease.
Red Mandarin essential oil	Toning, hydrating – a gentle oil often used for preventing or improving stretch marks.

Contraindications to treatment :

Your consultation form gives you a guide on conditions that,if present , mean either you cannot treat at all, can treat after the client has consulted their health care provider, or can treat with amendments to the procedure.

These conditions include:

Pregnancy – compression body wraps would not be an appropriate treatment at all, at any stage of pregnancy.

Circulatory disorders- including haemophilia, current thrombosis or blood clot, recent haemorrhage, clotting disorders,cardiac problems, varicose veins or phlebitis and uncontrolled high blood pressure would rule out tension wrapping . Rosemary essential oil is an ingredient in NSL balm and should not be used where there is significantly high blood pressure.

Slightly elevated, controlled hypertension may not be ruled out if a doctor or medical professional caring for the client sees no reason why they should not have the treatment.

Hypotension, or low blood pressure , would mean caution is required with positioning and you should advise the client to gradually and slowly rise from a lying position to seated, and then slowly from seated to standing to avoid dizziness.

Epilepsy: Rosemary essential oil is not suitable for use with people with epilepsy so treatment could not proceed.

Nut allergy : Shea butter is sourced from a tree nut and treatment should be avoided In those with nut allergy or sensitivity.

Kidney infection or disease: The juniper berry essential oil contained in NSL treatment balm is not suitable for use with those with kidney problems.

Diabetes: Tension wraps are often ruled out for those with this condition , especially where there is neuropathy (nerve damage meaning loss of sensation) which can occur with diabetes. Additionally, the process of lipolysis leads to the formation of ketones in the body. If there's insufficient insulin to help fuel the cells of the body, the build-up of ketones can become problematic for people with diabetes. Where the condition is controlled by diet, you may advise the client to check with their doctor before proceeding with treatment. Otherwise, treatment is not suitable.

Any condition causing loss of sensation in any area to be treated – for example, paralysis or Multiple Sclerosis – would rule out treatment as the client would be unable to feel whether the wrap was too tight or if there was a reaction to the product.

Infectious conditions : viral, bacterial or fungal - such as measles, shingles, influenza , scabies, impetigo – avoid treatment . This will not only prevent any worsening of the client's symptoms but will limit the possibility of the therapist contracting the condition. In some cases, some infectious conditions (eg warts or tinea) may be local contraindications rather than complete contraindications, provided they are not directly in the treatment area or can be worked around without detracting from the treatment.

Client under the influence of alcohol or drugs – do not treat.

Inflammation / swelling in the area to be treated – avoid treatment until resolved.

Unexplained or undiagnosed bruising, lumps or bumps: do not treat- without alarming the client, suggest they visit their GP to have this checked.

Bruising of known cause, cuts and abrasions: if it is possible to work around these and they are not severe then treatment can proceed.

Psoriasis or eczema: do not treat if skin is broken. Patch test of product is advisable before proceeding.

Sunburn: if mild, avoid body brushing and proceed to wrap. If moderate to severe, postpone treatment until skin has healed.

Contraceptive implant : take special care when working on the area around the implant . Do not massage directly over the area.

Cancer : the client should be advised to check with their consultant. If the client is undergoing chemotherapy or radiotherapy then treatment is not advised.

Recent surgery : dependent on the surgery , how long ago it was and whether healing is complete, it may be possible to proceed after consulting with the GP or consultant.

Contra-actions:

As with all treatments , there is a possibility of after effects or reactions during treatment, and these should be fully explained to the client .

During treatment:

Should any excessive reddening of the skin, itch or stinging become apparent, completely remove the product immediately with lukewarm water (in the case of an oil-based product, an unscented , mild liquid soap will help break down the oil molecules and should be applied neat and then swabbed with water) and bathe the affected area with cool water.

After treatment:

The client may feel **sleepy** as a result of treatment – ensure that they feel fully awake before they leave the premises. If they are driving, advise they keep a window open

,

Sometimes **headaches** or **mild nausea** occur after treatments- explain that this is as a result of the detoxification process and can be helped by carefully following aftercare advice and drinking enough water to help flush out the system.

Clients may feel **thirsty** – again, drinking water is advised. This may lead to increased **frequency of urination** as the body clears itself of waste products.

Occasionally **spots or blemishes** can occur – again this is a way of the body ridding itself of impurities.

Changes in sleep pattern – usually improvements – are sometimes noticed following a treatment.

Reassure the client that contra-actions do not always occur, but are generally mild and last no longer than 24- 48 hours if they do.

Treatment protocol

Step one: measuring

Ensure your measuring tape is straight and not twisted in order to give an accurate baseline measurement. You should mark the position of the tape for each area of the body measured so that when you measure again at the end of the session you are comparing like with like. Mark on the body at the top and bottom edges of the tape using a suitable pen such as a marker (so that the marks are not removed by product during treatment.

Points to measure are :

Left and right calf at fullest point

Left and right thigh – 2/3 of the way up from the knee

Hips: measure at the hip joint, ensuring the tape goes around rather than dropping below the buttocks

Lower abdomen : measure at the crest of the hipbone

Waist : measure at the narrowest point

Upper abdomen : measure around an inch below the ribcage.

Bust/ chest – measure at the fullest point.

Right and left upper arm : measure midway between shoulder and elbow

Right and left lower arm (if treating) – at fullest point (about a third of the way down from the elbow)

Step two: preparing the skin – exfoliation.

Body / dry brushing:

Dry brushing is a good way to exfoliate the skin and to boost the circulation, warming the area to be treated with the wrap balm. This aids absorption . Dry brushing is best carried out with natural bristle brushes, using very light pressure in brisk strokes on clean, dry skin. Brushing is always carried out toward the heart.

Firstly , establish with the client whether they are happy for you to include buttocks and the chest area in the brushing process.

Dry brushing can be carried out with the client standing up, or by turning the client on the couch midway through the process.

For the standard couch procedure:

.

Assist the client to lie prone (face down) on the couch. Drape with towels.

Legs:
- Undrape the right leg,.
- Work from knee to thigh in upward strokes,with light, brisk, overlapping brushing , and carry the movement onto the buttocks if your client has given approval to do this.
- To brush the inner thigh, stand at the client's hip, facing down the table, place both brushes on the inner thigh, and lightly pull with rhythmic strokes out towards the outer thigh.
- To brush the outer thigh, stand at the client's knee facing up the table, and briskly and lightly brush up the outer thigh to the hip with overlapping movements.
- Brush lightly and briskly from ankle to knee (avoid pressure over the popliteal cavity) use overlapping strokes as you work up ,one brush then the other, brushing in upwards strokes
- Finish brushing the legs by using long , light strokes from ankle all the way up to the hip.

- Cover the right leg
- Repeat on left leg.

Back:
- Undrape the back. Standing at the left side of the couch, place the brushes on the client's right side , and briskly and lightly pull the brushes inwards and upwards towards the spine. Alternate movements to cover the whole area.
- Move to the other side and repeat .
- Stand at the head of the table (slightly to one side) and place the brushes at the sacrum, sweeping lightly up to mid back with alternate movements.
- Sweep from shoulders to mid back (towards heart)
- Cover the back .

Backs of arms: sweep up from elbow to shoulder, then from wrist to elbow.

Turn client and place chest drape.and cover with towel.

Front of legs:
- Undrape the right leg, stand to the side of the couch and place brushes at inside of calf. Brush up and in towards mid line of leg, from ankle to knee taking care over the shin bone. Continue up the thigh .
- Stand at the foot of the couch and work up the middle of the leg from ankle to knee then knee to top of thigh with straight , alternate strokes upwards.
- Stand at the side of the couch and brush up the outside of the leg , ankle to knee, knee to hip.
- Cover leg and repeat on other side.

Abdomen brushing:
- Stand on the left side and place the brushes on the client's right side. Pull gently and briskly up towards the midline of the body
- Move to the top of the couch and pull brushes up the client's side in a straight line from hip to armpit, one side then the other.
- Move to the other side of the table and repeat the first move on the client's left side of the abdomen.

Breast/ chest area :

- Stand at the head of the table and brush from below the navel, pulling in a straight line between the breasts with overlapping strokes. To avoid the breast drape, simply lift the brush and "jump" over it.
- Brush from the armpit up and around the breast, ending at the upper part of the sternum. Again, "jump" the breast drape to keep the flow of the stroke.
- To finish the chest area, stand to one side of the massage table and brush across the upper chest from one shoulder to the other in a straight line.

Front of arms:

- Brush from elbow to shoulder
- Brush from fingers to elbow
- Finish arms with long sweeping stroked from fingers to shoulder.

Step three: Apply NSL treatment balm

With the client still on the couch, remove product from bowl with a clean spatula.

- Ask the client to bend their right leg and apply balm with sweeping strokes up the back of the calf and round to the front of the leg. Apply to front and then back of thigh with effleurage movements.

- Repeat on other leg.

- Undrape the client's abdomen and apply balm to the sides and abdomen using diamond effleurage movement. Massage balm into the hips and over lower ribs .

- Apply balm to arms with effleurage.. wrist to elbow, elbow to shoulder.

- Apply balm to décolletage, sweeping effleurage stroked from sternum out over triceps and round,

- Ask client to sit up and massage balm from base of spine to waist, base of spine to armpits, base of spine out over the shoulders. We work the upper back with effleurage, ensuring all the skin is covered.

Step 4 : Wrapping

DO NOT WRAP TOO TIGHTLY. *Wrap should never cut into the skin or impede circulation. Gently pull and stretch the wrap as you work. Pulling too tightly may rip the wrap material and cause your client discomfort, pain or injury*

Make sure the wrap is flat against the skin. Wrapping three times helps ensure good tension. Wrap slightly more loosely on the first pass, as this can help to prevent the rolling that can happen with film wrap , and more tightly on the second and third pass.
It is also useful to cross the wrap over in a saltire shape near the start of each part of the body, then again at the end, to help secure the wrap and ensure tension is maintained.

Help the client to get down from the couch..

- Using the smaller roll of wrap, start at the bottom of the calf and wind the wrap round and up the lower leg.

- Do not wrap tightly at the knees as the client will have to be able to bend them again to get back onto the couch.

- Continue wrapping up the thigh, criss-crossing the wrap from time to time to ensure it remains in place well.

- Wrap the other leg making sure tension is consistent.

- Wrap across the buttocks and around the hips with the larger wrap, making sure there are no gaps between the leg wrapping and the torso wrap. Continue up the body , and 'criss cross' the wrap over the shoulders.. Be careful not to wrap too tightly at the waist as this is where the wrap is most likely to roll down – see instructions in italics above to lessen the risk of this happening.

- Use the smaller roll of wrap to wrap the arms . If wrapping the lower arms, do not wrap too tightly at the elbows.

Assist the client onto the couch , cover warmly, and let the client relax as the wrap works.

At this point, you might wish to offer a foot or hand massage, or scalp massage if you have agreed this at treatment planning stage .Some salons will leave their client alone to rest as the wrap works, but a mini-treatment during this phase enhances the client experience and is in line with NSL's aim of an outstanding treatment and client care. Suggested routines for treatments will be included in our published manual.

At the end of the wrap processing time, remove the wrap and massage in any remaining product. Dispose of treatment waste and re-measure the client. Mark down the measurements in the appropriate section of the record , and calculate the total loss.

Let your client dress, while you wash your hands and get a glass of water for them to drink.

Go through aftercare advice with your client and arrange the next appointment.

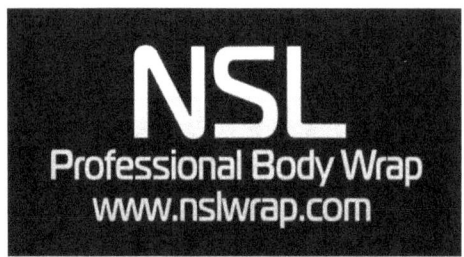

Aftercare advice for clients

For best results following your NSL wrap treatment, you should :

- Keep the product on for as long as possible to allow the active ingredients to keep working. If possible, don't shower or bathe till the following day .

- Drink between 8 – 10 glasses of water per day to help your body to flush out toxins.

- Avoid heat treatments, sunbathing or sunbeds for at least 24 hours after your treatment.

- Try to rest and relax immediately after your wrap

- Eat light meals for the remainder of the day .

- Avoid alcohol, tea, coffee and fizzy drinks.

Between treatments, it's helpful to:

- Increase the amount of fresh fruit and vegetables in your diet .

- Cut back on foods and cooking methods with a high fat content, added sugar and salt.

- Try to exercise daily – walking is ideal , and free!

- Use daily dry brushing to boost the circulation and improve skin condition.

- Apply the NSL scrub twice weekly to exfoliate and enhance treatment effects.

- Massage NSL contour oil into problem areas on a regular basis to boost the effects of the wrap. This will also hydrate and improve the appearance of your skin

We recommend a course of treatments for best results – ask your therapist for details.

Treatment Promotion

NSL wrap is perfect for anyone who is looking to lose inches, maybe kick starting a diet, trying to fit into a wedding dress or as part of your monthly body pampering.

Word of month: Word of month is a fantastic way to get the treatment known. People who have great results will tell their friends and soon you will have lots of free referrals. Perhaps you can have business cards to hand out with a code that will help you identify the particular client. The clients who has referred a certain amount of people could be offered a free treatment. Try to reward those who are helping you.

Social Media: Write interesting posts, have competitions for page members who 'like and share' your posts. Just one post to 100 Facebook followers can reach 1000's of their friends.

PR: Issue a press release to tell the media about your new treatment. Offer a complementary treatment to a local journalist / blogger in return for a review in their magazine / newspaper.

Advertising: Make sure you do not commit significant amounts of money in un-tested advertising. Try Google adwords but set a maximum budget. If your advertising budget is £30 per month set it at £1 per day, that way costs can not go higher.

Note: Make sure you have a website, even if it is only 1 page so that you can drive people to it to find our additional information and to book a course of treatments.

NSL posters and leaflets available.

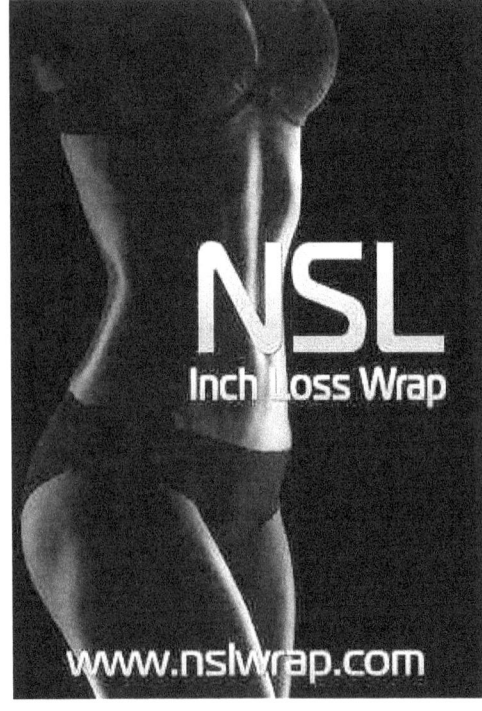 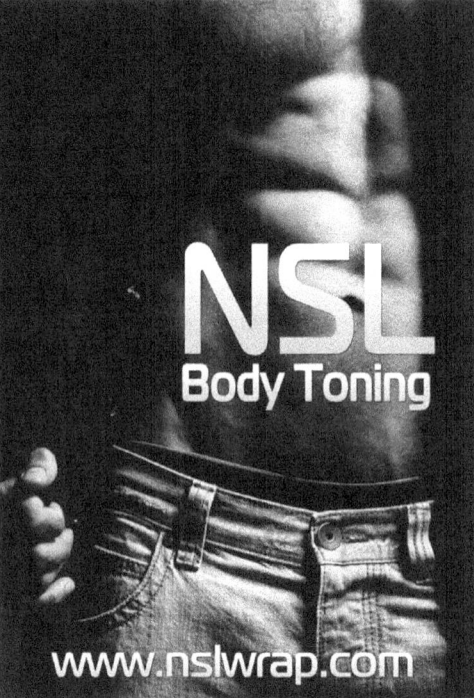

Simple Black and White NSL Posters

Summer promotion: We decided this summer instead of competing with other brands we would highlight our unique selling point. This advert sells the skincare side of the treatment with the inch loss as a bonus!

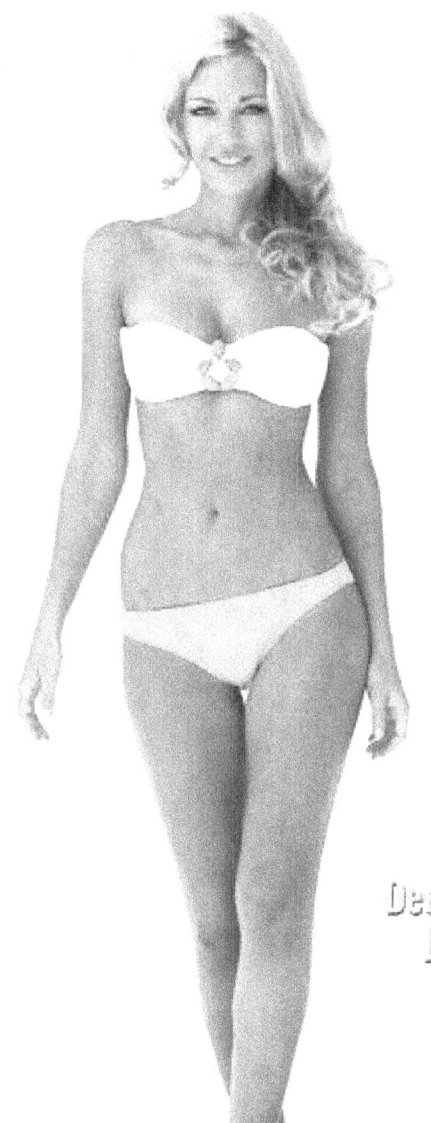

NSL

NSL Wrap - Will leave your skin super soft and cared for, helps stretch marks.

Is your body ready for summer?

Deeply moisturing and nourishing Luxurious spa and salon only body treatment.

Inch loss results are part of this treatment, your clothes may fit better and you may appear slimmer. 100% of clients in our trial experienced inch loss.

www.nslwrap.com

NSL Facial, a 6 in 1 facial treatment. If interested in finding out about this complementary treatment please email info@ctacademy.co.uk

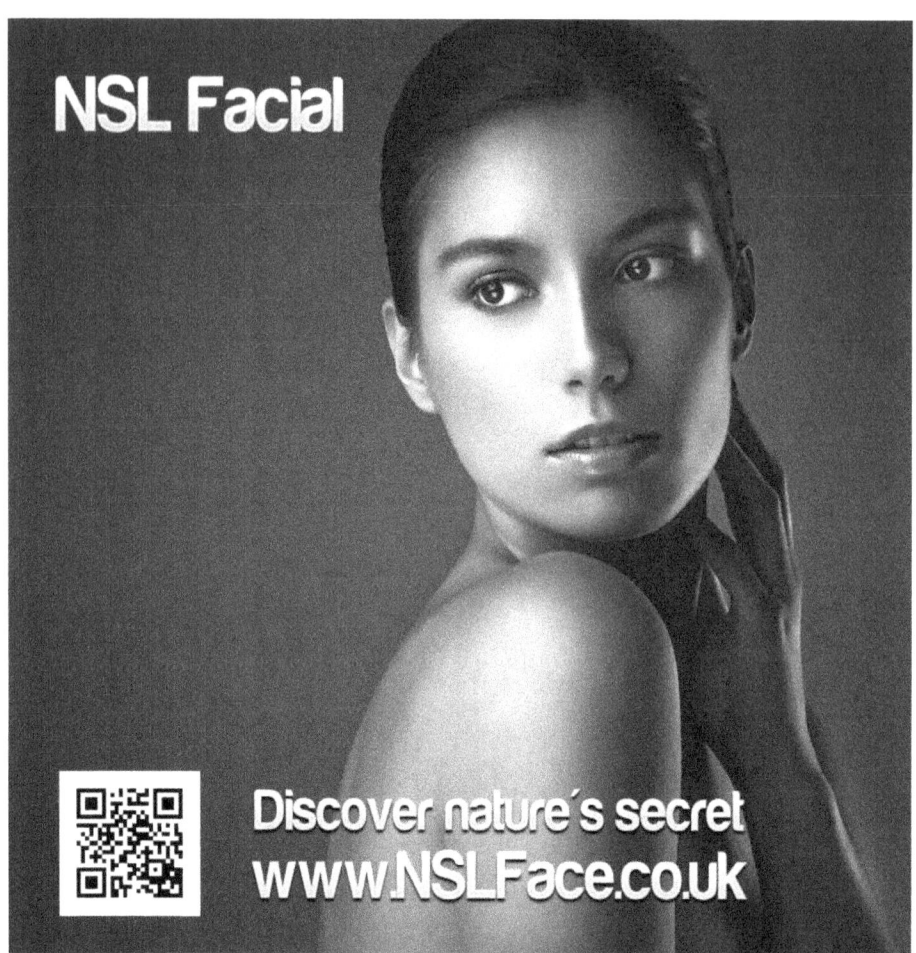

If you like this book you may also like...

Lash Masters, Nail Masters, Beauty Masters, Flirties A-Z of Lash Enhancements.

Available from Amazon.

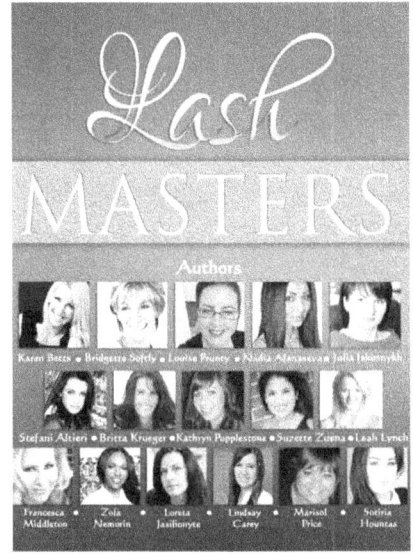

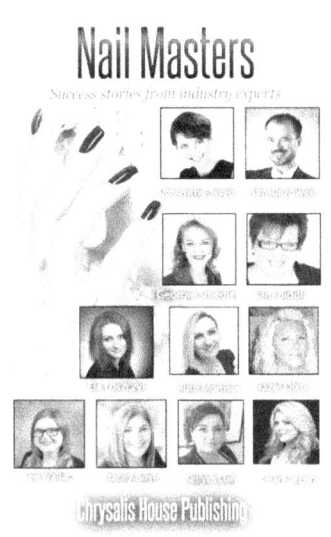

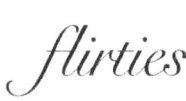

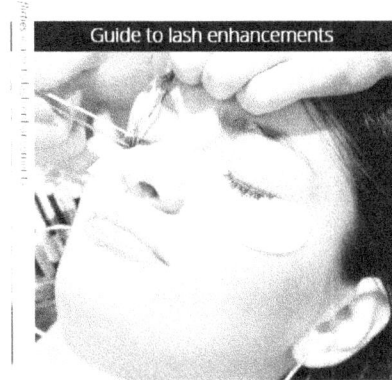

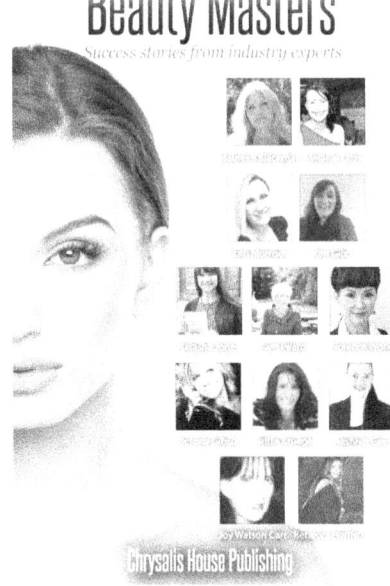